I0781791

SARDINIAN DIET PLAN COOK BOOK

The Sardinian Diet: Recipes for Longevity and Foods that Enhance Health and Longevity

REX LEWIS

Copyright © 2024 by REX LEWIS

All Rights Reserved.

Table of Contents

Introduction

The Sardinian diet is commonly linked to the customary eating habits of the inhabitants of Sardinia, an Italian island located in the Mediterranean Sea. Sardinia has garnered recognition for its notable prevalence of centenarians—individuals who reach the age of 100 or beyond—and scientists have examined the lifestyle and dietary practices of the Sardinian populace in order to comprehend the elements that contribute to their longevity.

The Sardinian diet and lifestyle encompass several important elements:

• The Sardinian diet is a specific version of the Mediterranean diet, known for its emphasis on consuming abundant quantities of fruits, vegetables, legumes, whole grains, nuts, and olive oil.

• Given the island's maritime position, fish and seafood are important constituents of the cuisine.

• **Plant-Based Focus:** Sardinians have a long-standing practice of consuming a diverse range of fruits and vegetables that are cultivated locally, which supply them with crucial vitamins, minerals, and antioxidants.

• Legumes, such as beans and lentils, are prevalent in their diet and provide a substantial amount of protein and fiber.

• Whole grains, such as barley and wheat, are fundamental components of the Sardinian diet. These grains offer long-lasting energy and are rich in dietary fiber.

• **Dairy Products:** Sardinians frequently partake in the consumption of dairy products, including sheep's milk and cheese. Pecorino cheese, derived from the milk of sheep, is a widely favored option that boasts a high content of calcium and beneficial fats.

• **Wine Consumption:** Moderate wine consumption, particularly red wine, is an integral aspect of the Sardinian way of life. Red wine includes antioxidants, specifically resveratrol, that may provide health advantages.

• **Restricted Meat Consumption:** Sardinians usually consume meat in reduced proportions compared to other Western cuisines, however it is nevertheless part of their diet. Lean meats, such as lamb and hog, are frequently eaten.

• **Physical Exercise:** Furthermore, the Sardinian way of life incorporates consistent engagement in physical exercise, in addition to their nutritional choices. A significant number of Sardinians partake in regular physical activities, including walking, gardening, and manual labor.

• **Social and Community links:** The social dimension of meals and robust community links are fundamental to the Sardinian way of life. Partaking in communal meals with loved ones is a prevalent custom that fosters a feeling of togetherness and enhances emotional welfare.

Studies indicate that the amalgamation of these nutritional and behavioral elements plays a role in the well-being and extended lifespan observed in the population of Sardinia. It is important to acknowledge that although diet is a crucial influence, other aspects of lifestyle, such as heredity and environmental variables, also contribute to the overall health of the community.

CHAPTER ONE
Sardinia: A Culinary and Cultural Overview

Sardinia, the second-largest island in the Mediterranean Sea, possesses a diverse and valuable culinary and cultural legacy. The island's historical, geographical, and traditional aspects have greatly shaped its distinct cuisine and way of living. Below is a comprehensive overview of the culinary and cultural aspects of Sardinia:

Culinary Summary:

• The cuisine of Sardinia is heavily influenced by the Mediterranean diet, which places a strong emphasis on using fresh, locally sourced ingredients such as olive oil, fruits, vegetables, and seafood.

• **Pasta and Bread:** Malloreddus, a variety of pasta from Sardinia, is a commonly enjoyed option, frequently accompanied by a variety of sauces.

• Pane Carasau, a traditional Sardinian flatbread, is extensively consumed. The product is slender, crunchy, and has a prolonged period of freshness, which makes it well-suited for the challenging landscape of the island.

• **Cheeses:** Sardinia is famous for its cheese manufacturing. Pecorino cheese, derived from the milk of sheep, is a fundamental and essential food item. Popular varieties include Pecorino Sardo and Fiore Sardo.

• Casu Marzu, a traditional cheese from Sardinia, is renowned for its distinctive production method that involves the use of live insect larvae.

• Seafood is an important component of Sardinian cuisine due to its coastal location. Common culinary offerings include grilled fish, seafood stews, and dishes that prominently showcase locally sourced catches.

• Culurgiones are traditional Sardinian dumplings that are typically stuffed with ingredients such as potatoes, mint, and cheese. They are commonly served with a tomato or meat sauce.

- **Meat Dishes:** Lamb, hog, and game meats are widely utilized in Sardinian cuisine. Roast suckling pig (porceddu) is a classic delicacy.

- **Sweets & Desserts:** Seadas, a dessert pastry, is a delicacy of Sardinia. It is loaded with cheese and generally drizzled with honey.

- Amaretti cookies, made with almonds, are another beloved sweet delicacy.

Cultural Overview:

1. **Nuragic Civilization:** Sardinia is home to the ancient Nuragic civilization, famed for its remarkable stone constructions called Nuraghes. These ancient ruins are dispersed over

the island and constitute a vital element of Sardinia's cultural heritage.

2. Language: Sardinian, a Romance language, is spoken alongside Italian. The island's linguistic diversity reflects its unique cultural identity.

3. Festivals and Traditions: Sardinians celebrate many traditional festivals, generally highlighted by colorful processions, music, and dancing. The Cavalcata Sarda is a famous equestrian event conducted in Sassari.

• The Mamuthones and Issohadores Carnival in Mamoiada incorporates historic mask-wearing practices.

4. Craftsmanship: Sardinia is famed for its traditional crafts, including handwoven textiles, ceramics, and filigree jewelry. Villages like Samugheo are renowned for their artisanal items.

5. Music and Dance: Traditional Sardinian music, including the use of the launeddas (triple-reeded pipes), and dance, such as the ballu tundu, play a crucial role in local celebrations and cultural gatherings.

6. The culture of Sardinia has been significantly influenced by the historical practice of shepherding. The terrain is scattered with shelters used by shepherds, and the rural way of life is honored through diverse cultural manifestations.

The gastronomic and cultural abundance of Sardinia can be attributed to a blend of historical influences, geographical elements, and the islanders' determination to uphold their traditions. When people visit Sardinia, they frequently experience a rich assortment of tastes and traditions that showcase the island's distinct character.

How the Sardinian Diet Is Based on Science

Researchers are interested in the science of the Sardinian cuisine because of its possible health benefits, particularly in increasing longevity. According to research, there are a number of components that work together to make the diet healthy. Although diet does play a part, other lifestyle choices, heredity, and environmental factors also contribute to the general well-being and longevity seen in Sardinian populations. Some important parts of the Sardinian diet's scientific basis are as follows:

- Elements of the Mediterranean Diet:
- The health benefits of the Mediterranean diet have been the subject of substantial research, and the Sardinian diet shares many of its features. A wide variety of nutrients and antioxidants are provided by the diet's focus on fresh produce, whole grains, beans, almonds, olive oil, and seafood.

- Olive oil is full of polyphenols and monounsaturated fats; it is an essential part of the Sardinian diet. These ingredients offer anti-inflammatory and cardiovascular health benefits.

- A high intake of antioxidants is provided by the Sardinian diet's abundance of fruits, vegetables, and nuts. By scavenging harmful free radicals, these chemicals may lessen the effects of oxidative stress and inflammation.

4. Sardinian Diet and Omega-3 Fatty Acids: Sardinians get more omega-3 fatty acids from their fish consumption. Omega-3 fatty acids lower the risk of cardiovascular disease and other cardiovascular complications.

5. Intake of Wine: Some health benefits have been linked to moderate intake of red wine, which is widespread in Sardinia. Resveratrol is one of several polyphenols found in red wine that may have anti-inflammatory and antioxidant properties.

6. Plant-Based Proteins: Legumes and plant-based proteins play a big role in the diet and help keep nutrients in check. Lower prevalence of certain chronic diseases are just one of the many health benefits associated with plant-based diets.

7. Moderate Meat Consumption: Lean meats, such as lamb and pork, make up a smaller portion of the typical Sardinian diet. Guidelines for improving heart health and decreasing consumption of saturated fat are congruent with this feature.

8. Dietary Fiber-Rich Whole Grains: Cereals and wheat are examples of whole grains that are rich in fiber. In addition to reducing the risk of cardiovascular disease and type 2 diabetes, fiber aids digestion.

9. Sardinian Cheese and Sheep's Milk: Sardinians get their calcium and other nutrients from the dairy products made from sheep. Cheesemaking, which involves fermentation, may potentially have beneficial effects on digestive health.

10. Lifestyle Factors: Supplementing a healthy diet with other aspects of Sardinian culture, like as frequent exercise, close friendships, and a strong feeling of community, is said to be the most important thing one can do to promote health and longevity.

Individual health outcomes are complicated and affected by numerous factors; nonetheless, research indicates that the Sardinian diet could be a contributing factor to the observed community longevity. Also, our current scientific understanding of these eating behaviors is always expanding, and new studies are always trying to pin down the exact mechanisms at work.

CHAPTER TWO
Key Principles of the Sardinian Diet

The Sardinian cuisine is distinguished by a number of fundamental principles that contribute to its possible health advantages and the long lifespan observed in the population. Although individual dietary choices may differ, the traditional Sardinian cuisine is typically characterized by the following principles:

1. Plant-Based Focus: The diet mostly consists of plant-based foods, such as fruits, vegetables, legumes, nuts, and whole grains. These foods offer a diverse range of vitamins, minerals, antioxidants, and dietary fiber.

2. Olive Oil as the Main Fat Source: Olive oil, especially extra virgin olive oil, is the predominant fat source in the Sardinian diet. The presence of monounsaturated fats and polyphenols in it promotes cardiovascular well-being and has anti-inflammatory properties.

3. Sardinians have a high intake of a diverse range of fresh, locally sourced fruits and vegetables. These foods are abundant in vitamins, minerals, and antioxidants, which promote overall health and well-being.

4. Fish and Seafood: Fish and seafood, particularly those sourced from the Mediterranean Sea, serve as significant protein providers. In addition, they provide omega-3 fatty acids, which are recognized for their positive effects on the cardiovascular system.

5. Moderate Wine Consumption: Red wine is consumed in moderation as a component of the Sardinian lifestyle. Consuming red wine in moderate amounts can provide certain health advantages because of its polyphenol composition, which includes resveratrol.

6. Restricted Consumption of Red Meat: Sardinians traditionally consume lesser quantities of red meat, with a preference for leaner alternatives such as lamb and pork.

Sheep's milk and cheese, namely Pecorino cheese, are frequently consumed in the Sardinian cuisine. These dairy products offer vital minerals, including calcium and protein.

8. Whole Grains: Whole grains such as barley and wheat are essential foods that offer complex carbs, fiber, and long-lasting energy.

9. Herbs and spices are utilized to enhance the taste of dishes, hence decreasing the need for excessive salt or unhealthy condiments. This enhances the overall nutritional quality of the diet.

10. Cultural and Social Aspects: Meals are frequently enjoyed in the company of family and friends, highlighting the social and cultural importance of food. The collective nature of meals enhances a feeling of camaraderie and overall welfare.

11. Physical Activity: The traditional Sardinian lifestyle involves frequent physical activity, which is generally linked to outdoor activities, farming, and manual labor. Physical activity is seen as essential for overall well-being.

12. The Sardinian diet is shaped by the seasonal and local availability of ingredients. This encourages the intake of fresh, locally obtained foods with less processing.

It is crucial to acknowledge that these principles serve as a broad characterization of the conventional Sardinian diet, and individual dietary habits may differ. In addition, although diet is an important influence, other lifestyle choices, genetics, and environmental variables also contribute to the health and long lifespan found in Sardinian communities.

Sardinian Superfoods

The traditional Sardinian diet includes several nutrient-dense foods that are often considered "superfoods" due to their rich nutritional profiles and potential health benefits. Here are some Sardinian superfoods commonly included in the island's traditional cuisine:

Pecorino Cheese:

• Pecorino cheese, made from sheep's milk, is a staple in Sardinian cuisine. It is rich in protein, calcium, and essential fatty acids. The fermentation process involved in cheese production also contributes to the presence of probiotics, promoting gut health.

Extra Virgin Olive Oil:

• Extra virgin olive oil is a key component of the Sardinian diet. It is a source of monounsaturated fats and polyphenols, which have been associated with cardiovascular health and anti-inflammatory effects.

Fava Beans:

• Fava beans are a common legume in Sardinian dishes. They are high in protein, fiber, and various vitamins and minerals, contributing to a well-rounded nutrient profile.

Barley:

• Barley is a staple whole grain in Sardinia, often used in soups and stews. It is a good source of dietary fiber, vitamins, and minerals, providing sustained energy and supporting digestive health.

Cannonau Wine:

• Cannonau wine, a red wine produced in Sardinia, has gained attention for its potential health benefits. It is made from the Cannonau grape, which has a high concentration of antioxidants, including resveratrol.

Carasau Bread:

• Carasau, or carta da musica, is a traditional Sardinian flatbread. It is low in fat, rich in carbohydrates, and has a long shelf life. The thin, crisp bread is often served with various toppings or used in soups.

Mediterranean Fish:

• Sardinians have access to a variety of fresh fish and seafood from the Mediterranean Sea. Fatty fish, such as mackerel and sardines, are rich in omega-3 fatty acids, contributing to heart health.

Tomatoes:

• Tomatoes are a common ingredient in Sardinian cuisine, providing vitamins, minerals, and antioxidants. They are often used in sauces, salads, and various dishes.

Myrtle Berries:

• Myrtle berries are used in Sardinian cuisine to make a traditional liqueur called "Mirto." The berries are rich in antioxidants and have been associated with potential health benefits.

Malloreddus Pasta:

• Malloreddus, a type of Sardinian pasta, is often made from semolina flour. While not a superfood in the traditional sense, it is a local specialty and a source of carbohydrates.

It's important to note that the term "superfood" is not a scientific classification, and the health benefits of these foods are best understood as part of a balanced and diverse diet. The combination of these nutrient-dense foods, along with the overall dietary and lifestyle patterns of Sardinia, contributes to the potential

health advantages observed in the
population.

CHAPTER THREE
Meal Planning and Recipes

Meal planning based on the principles of the Sardinian diet can be a flavorful and nutritious way to incorporate the key elements of this traditional eating pattern into your routine. Here's a sample day of meal ideas inspired by the Sardinian diet:

Breakfast:

Fruit and Nut Yogurt Parfait:

- Greek yogurt with a drizzle of local honey.
- Fresh Sardinian fruits such as figs or citrus segments.

- Sprinkle with chopped nuts (almonds, walnuts, or hazelnuts).

Mid-Morning Snack:

Whole Grain Crackers with Pecorino Cheese:

- Whole grain crackers or carasau bread.
- Slices of Pecorino cheese.
- A handful of grapes or cherry tomatoes.

Lunch:

Malloreddus Pasta with Tomato Sauce and Vegetables:

- Malloreddus pasta made from durum wheat semolina.

- Tomato sauce with garlic, onions, and Sardinian tomatoes.

- Include vegetables such as zucchini, eggplant, and bell peppers.

- Drizzle with extra virgin olive oil.

- A side salad with mixed greens, olives, and a simple olive oil and lemon dressing.

Afternoon Snack:

Fresh Fruit Smoothie:

- Blend Sardinian berries (like myrtle berries or local berries) with banana.

- Add a spoonful of Greek yogurt or almond milk for creaminess.

- Optional: a touch of local honey.

Dinner:

Grilled Fish with Herbs:

- Fresh Mediterranean fish like sea bass or sardines, seasoned with a mixture of fresh herbs (rosemary, thyme, oregano).
- Served with a side of roasted or steamed seasonal vegetables (broccoli, carrots, or asparagus).
- Quinoa or barley pilaf seasoned with olive oil and lemon.

Dessert:

Seadas:

- Homemade seadas, a traditional Sardinian dessert.

- Prepare a thin pastry filled with pecorino cheese, lemon zest, and a touch of honey.

- Fry until golden and drizzle with more honey.

- Tips for Sardinian-Inspired Meal Planning:

Local and Seasonal Ingredients:

• Emphasize locally sourced and seasonal ingredients to capture the freshness and flavors of Sardinian cuisine.

Olive Oil as a Key Ingredient:

• Use extra virgin olive oil in salad dressings, for sautéing, and as a finishing touch for added flavor.

Variety of Fruits and Vegetables:

• Incorporate a colorful array of fruits and vegetables to ensure a diverse range of nutrients.

Lean Proteins:

• Include fish, lean meats (such as lamb or pork in moderation), and plant-based proteins like legumes in your meals.

Whole Grains:

• Opt for whole grains like barley, quinoa, or whole wheat pasta for a good source of fiber and nutrients.

Moderate Wine Consumption:

• If you choose to consume alcohol, consider incorporating a glass of red wine with your meals, in moderation.

Social Dining:

• Enjoy meals with family and friends to promote a sense of community and well-being.

Remember to adapt these meal ideas to your individual preferences, dietary needs, and portion sizes. The Sardinian diet is not about strict rules but rather a balanced and enjoyable approach to eating that prioritizes whole, nutrient-dense foods.

Factors That Influence One's Way of Life

The Sardinian way of life is a vital factor in the overall well-being and extended life expectancy found in the people. In addition to eating choices, other lifestyle aspects contribute to the overall well-being of the Sardinian population. The Sardinian way of life is characterized by several fundamental lifestyle factors:

1. Physical Activity: Traditional Sardinian lives frequently incorporate consistent engagement in physical activities. Engaging in daily activities such as walking, gardening, and manual labor fosters an active lifestyle, which enhances cardiovascular health and general well-being.

2. Outdoor Living: The favorable weather conditions and picturesque surroundings of the island promote engagement in outdoor pursuits. Residents frequently engage in outdoor activities, immersing themselves in nature, which can positively impact their mental well-being and alleviate stress.

3. Sardinian societies prioritize and highly appreciate social interactions and familial relationships. Consistent social engagements, collective endeavors, and assistance systems enhance emotional wellness and foster a feeling of inclusion.

4. Cultural Practices and Celebrations: Engaging in customary cultural practices, festivals, and celebrations is a prevalent characteristic of life in Sardinia. These events offer chances for social interaction, promoting a robust sense of community.

5. Work-Life Balance: The traditional Sardinian culture frequently prioritizes maintaining a harmonious equilibrium between work and leisure activities. This equilibrium can potentially lead to reduced levels of stress and enhanced mental well-being.

6. Sardinians possess a strong affinity for nature, which is seen in their engagement with agricultural methods, participation in outdoor activities, and their genuine admiration for the island's natural splendor. This relationship is linked to psychological well-being and a feeling of calmness.

7. Sardinian communities frequently preserve a profound reverence for tradition and cultural history. This level of respect creates a feeling of selfhood and consistency, promoting a secure and stabilizing atmosphere.

8. Limited Exposure to Contemporary Stressors: In certain rural regions of Sardinia, inhabitants may have restricted exposure to the stressors associated with modern urban living. This could perhaps lead to a more tranquil way of life and reduced levels of persistent stress.

9. The notion of "active aging" is widely embraced in Sardinia, where a significant number of elderly adults maintain their physical activity levels and actively participate in community affairs. Active aging is linked to improved quality of life and increased longevity.

10. Sardinian communities frequently integrate natural and traditional healing practices into their way of life. This may encompass the utilization of indigenous herbs, flora, and therapeutic solutions, hence promoting comprehensive wellness.

11. Decreased prevalence of tobacco use:In comparison to numerous other regions, Sardinia has comparatively low prevalence of smoking. Restricting tobacco consumption is a favorable aspect of one's lifestyle that enhances cardiovascular and respiratory well-being.

It is critical to acknowledge that although lifestyle factors are significant, genetics and environmental factors also contribute to the observed health outcomes in Sardinia. The Sardinian way of life is characterized by a combination of a well-rounded diet, regular physical activity, meaningful social relationships, and cultural traditions,

all of which contribute to its distinct
and health-enhancing qualities.

CHAPTER FOUR
Incorporating Sardinian Diet Principles into Your Life

Incorporating the principles of the Sardinian diet into your life can be a flavorful and healthful approach to eating. Here are some practical tips to help you embrace the Sardinian diet principles:

Prioritize Plant-Based Foods:

• Make fruits, vegetables, legumes, and whole grains the foundation of your meals. Aim to fill at least half your plate with these nutrient-dense, plant-based options.

Use Extra Virgin Olive Oil:

• Use extra virgin olive oil as your primary source of fat for cooking and dressing salads. It not only adds a rich flavor but also provides heart-healthy monounsaturated fats.

Incorporate Seafood:

• Include fish and seafood in your diet, especially varieties rich in omega-3 fatty acids. Aim for at least two servings of fatty fish per week, such as salmon, mackerel, or sardines.

Choose Lean Proteins:

• When consuming meat, opt for lean options like poultry or lean cuts of lamb or pork. Consider incorporating more plant-based protein sources like legumes and nuts.

Enjoy Whole Grains:

• Replace refined grains with whole grains like barley, quinoa, whole wheat, and oats. These grains provide more fiber, vitamins, and minerals.

Moderate Wine Consumption:

• If you choose to drink alcohol, particularly wine, do so in moderation. One glass of red wine per day with meals is a common practice in the Sardinian diet.

Include Local and Seasonal Ingredients:

• Embrace local and seasonal produce to enhance the freshness and flavor of your meals. Visit local farmers' markets to explore and support regional offerings.

Experiment with Sardinian Recipes:

• Try your hand at preparing traditional Sardinian dishes like Malloreddus pasta, seadas, or grilled fish with Sardinian herbs. Experimenting with these recipes can be a fun way to immerse yourself in the culinary traditions.

Prioritize Social Dining:

• Embrace the social aspect of meals. Share meals with family and friends, creating a sense of community and fostering positive connections.

Stay Active:

• Incorporate regular physical activity into your routine. Whether it's walking, gardening, or engaging in outdoor activities, staying active is a fundamental aspect of the Sardinian lifestyle.

Cultivate a Relaxed Environment:

• Foster a relaxed mealtime environment. Take time to savor and enjoy your meals, avoiding rushed or stressful eating situations.

Connect with Nature:

• Spend time outdoors, appreciating nature and incorporating activities like hiking, biking, or gardening into your routine.

Explore Local Herbs and Spices:

• Experiment with local herbs and spices to add flavor to your dishes. Sardinian cuisine often incorporates herbs like rosemary, thyme, and oregano.

Practice Portion Control:

• Pay attention to portion sizes. Sardinians traditionally practice moderation in their servings, which contributes to a balanced and healthful approach to eating.

Embrace the Mediterranean Lifestyle:

• Consider adopting other Mediterranean lifestyle practices, such as engaging in social activities, getting sufficient rest, and managing stress through relaxation techniques.

Remember that the key to a sustainable and healthful lifestyle is to find a balance that works for you. Gradually incorporating these principles into your routine can lead to positive changes in your overall well-being.

Conclusion

Ultimately, the Sardinian diet and lifestyle provide a comprehensive approach to promoting health and longevity that goes beyond mere culinary decisions. The Sardinian lifestyle is founded on the ideas of the Mediterranean diet, which focuses on plant-based foods, olive oil, lean proteins, and a balanced, communal approach to meals. The utilization of indigenous and timely constituents, coupled with a dedication to physical exertion, communal bonds, and an affiliation with the natural environment, enhances the holistic welfare of the inhabitants of Sardinia.

Although the Sardinian cuisine has been linked to positive health effects and long life, it is important to acknowledge that lifestyle choices, genetic variables, and the surrounding environment all contribute to determining an individual's health outcomes. Embracing the principles of the Sardinian diet can provide a framework for a healthy and pleasurable way of life. However, it is important to take into account personal tastes, cultural background, and specific health requirements.

By adopting aspects of the Sardinian lifestyle, people can discover delectable and nutritious cuisine, participate in consistent exercise, value interpersonal relationships, and foster a more laid-back approach to daily existence. Whether you choose to include particular Sardinian foods in your cooking or simply embrace the general concepts of a Mediterranean diet, the objective is to establish a sustainable and pleasurable approach to eating and living that enhances overall health and well-being.

THE END